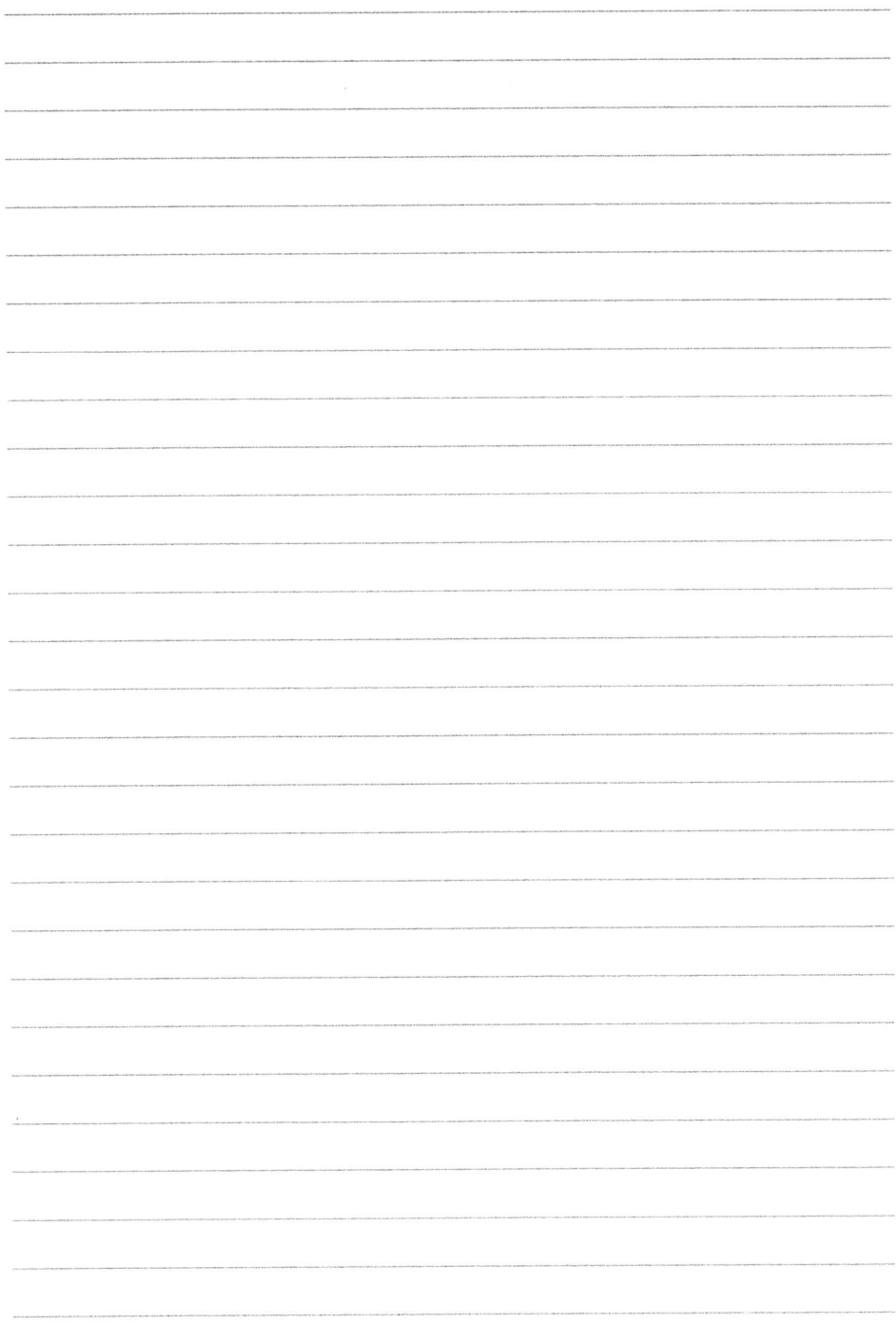

First Responder Nurse Journal Notebook
Caring Is What We Do: First Responder Journal Series
Gift Book Ideas For Nurses
Paperback ISBN: 978-1-989733-45-5
Copyright Dunhill Clare Publishing 2020
All Rights Reserved. Cover Design by Sharon Purtill